BREATHING FOR TWO

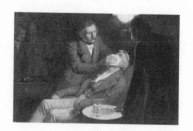

WOLF PASCOE

Tinderbox Books

1315 Malcolm Ave., Los Angeles, CA 90024

676 Darlington Road, Atlanta, GA 30305

ISBN: 1939803012

ISBN-13: 978-1-939803-01-6

ISBN (ebook): 978-1-939803-00-9

Library of Congress (LCCN): 2013934862

For Nick and Nora

CONTENTS

BREATHING FOR TWO

PROLOGUE

WHEN I WAS in medical school, I heard about a curious malady called Ondine's curse. It was a breathing disorder, and the professor had casually mentioned it during a lecture on the mechanics of breathing—an afterthought, more or less.

"Who was Ondine?" someone asked.

The professor didn't know.

Who coined the name?

It was an anesthesiologist who had observed it in patients with injuries to the respiratory center—the part of the brain that controls breathing.

"What's the cure?" someone else said.

"There isn't one."

You hear about many disorders when you're in medical school, of course. Some you think about a lot. Some you even begin to think you have, but usually you get over it.

Ondine's curse is this: during sleep, the body forgets to breathe.

Ondine was a water nymph who fell in love with a man. It's dangerous business for a nymph to get involved with a mortal, for if she has a child by him she loses her immortality. This happened to Ondine, who was content with her fate until she discovered her husband sleeping with another woman.

Ondine woke her unlucky spouse with her curse: *You promised faithfulness with every breath. Let it be done. Should you ever fall asleep again, you shall not breathe.*

Was ever revenge more poetically correct?

Fortunately, permanent ruin of the respiratory center is rare. I don't have Ondine's curse, and neither do you, probably, if you're reading this. On the other hand, I encounter a temporary form of Ondine's curse every day in surgery, where, as an anesthesiologist, I must routinely interrupt normal breathing in order to make surgery possible. An anesthesiologist, you might say, is the Ondine of the operating room.

Let me set the scene.

You're an observer in a modern OR. Even though there are no windows, you know the sun hasn't yet risen. A middle-aged woman lies awake on the table.

A nondescript but intense man in scrubs speaks intimately into her ear. The man isn't acting as you imagine a surgeon would—he seems oblivious to the surgical paraphernalia in the room.

You see the man remove an empty syringe from an

injection port and flick the intravenous line with the back of his hand. The woman's eyes flutter and close. One hand, with which she'd been tapping a sort of rhythm on her thigh, goes limp. Her chest stops rising and falling.

One moment the woman was there, and now she's gone. You're not sure, exactly, what has just happened.

The nurses pay no attention, either to the woman or the man. Nothing noteworthy here, they seem to say. They go about their business, talking quietly, wheeling trays around, opening packs of instruments.

The man lifts a strange, plastic cone off the woman's face —when did it get there? He pivots and retrieves a bizarre flashlight from an adjacent cart, and begins looking in the woman's mouth. You notice the gas machine at the man's side, a cascade of glass columns, porcelain knobs and metal conduits too complex to fathom. The machine makes a rushing sound and the woman's chest rises and falls.

The machine is breathing for her.

The man tapes the woman's eyes closed, picks up the chart, and starts writing. The woman is inert, insensible. Her transformation into surgical tissue has taken less than a minute.

ð ð ð

It took me many thousands of hours to become the man

in that vignette. I'm still becoming him.

It's been said that anesthesiologists are the last clinical generalists. They need, apart from expertise in anesthesia, physiology, anatomy, and pharmacology, a working grasp of most other medical disciplines. Obstetrics, cardiology, pediatrics, radiology, neurology, pulmonology, endocrinology —the list, including the surgical specialties, goes on.

All that is true, and a lot of learning it is. But that isn't the heart of it. The warp and woof of anesthesia is something strange, an essence different from other fields of medicine, the realization of which has come to me slowly over time, obvious only in retrospect.

In all other clinical specialties, surgical and medical, the doctor's object is to prevent illness when possible; if not to prevent, then to cure; if not to cure, then to alleviate.

But in anesthesia, the object is to incapacitate.

Incapacitate, incapacitated. As in no thought, no awareness, no memory, no response, no movement, no breath. The anesthetist prevents no disorder, cures no affliction, and makes better no illness. His peculiar occupation is to turn a living soul into tissue.

I've been coming to grips with this strangeness in my profession for many years. I've groped for metaphors to express it. My favorite is the night sea journey. It goes like this:

I'm a boatman sailing across a body of water, and the

patient is my sleeping passenger. It's night. If we make it to the other side, a change in the patient, a change that involves healing, takes place. But I don't directly participate in that. My job is to keep the boat moving.

Crossing the dark water poses many dangers: storms and headwinds, rocks and whirlpools, even dragons. When the boat leaks, I undertake repairs. When it veers off course, I must find the way again. None of this is much fun. A lot of it is harrowing. Hours of boredom, moments of panic, as they say.

The boatman's journey is a romantic metaphor I like telling. I think of myself as the custodian of that craft and its precious cargo, sustaining a ritual of healing. But uppermost in my mind is the harrowing part of being a boatman.

Of all the dangers in an operating room, the most harrowing involves Ondine's curse (I mentioned before that the anesthesiologist routinely must interrupt normal breathing). The anesthesiologist therefore routinely faces a harrowing question: *what do you do with a body that can't breathe?*

The strangeness an anesthetist can experience—the strangeness I experience—comes from this: from being both Ondine's instrument and antidote; from the need both to steal breath from my patient and then to restore it. This adds a subtle wrinkle to the metaphor of the boatman: the dangers of the journey come not only from outside, but from the boatman himself.

In my own case, enacting this little drama has taken a toll over time. To be sure, the journey changes the patient. But it also changes me.

One

Breathing lessons

IN THE FRESHMAN year of my anesthesia residency, I was given a lesson in breathing by a patient whom I'll call Otto. Anesthesia residencies come replete with breathing lessons, but Otto was also teaching humility that day, a subject absent from the formal anesthesia curriculum.

A doctor gets humility not from curricula but from his patients. I acquired a truckload of humility the day I met Otto, and the truck has only gotten larger since.

Otto was undergoing a cystoscopy, a look inside the bladder performed by passing a thin viewing scope through the urethra. There is no incision in such a procedure.

Generally, you don't need anything fancy to support a patient's breathing while giving anesthesia during a cystoscopy. As the patient passes from wakefulness into unconsciousness you can let him continue to breathe for

1

himself.

In Otto's case, I strapped a rubber anesthesia mask over his mouth and nose to make an airtight seal against his skin, and delivered through the mask an appropriate combination of oxygen and anesthetic gas. In principle, what I did was essentially what the Boston dentist, William Thomas Green Morton, had done during the first public demonstration of ether anesthesia in 1846.

The modern anesthesia face mask is a hollow cone of rubber or plastic. It's like the oxygen mask that drops down from above a passenger's head on an airplane, though it's more substantially built. The base is malleable and cushioned by a ring of air, a sort of inner tube. The mask is shaped to fit around the nose and mouth; with a bit of pressure, it seals against the skin. The top of the mask connects to a source of anesthetic vapor and oxygen.

Readers of a certain age may remember the TV series, *Marcus Welby, M.D.*, which began each week with Dr. Welby lowering a black anesthesia mask down over the camera lens. In those days, apparently, the family doctor did everything.

The anesthesia machine—the "cascade of glass columns, porcelain knobs and metal conduits" I described previously—is the gas delivery system. The machine connects to an oxygen tank and directs the flow of oxygen from the tank through a vaporizer where the oxygen mixes with anesthesia gas. The mixture passes out of the machine through plastic tubing ("anesthesia hose") that connects to the face mask.

The patient breathes the mixture.

Gas leaving the anesthesia machine actually flows through the anesthesia tubing in a circle—in fact it's called the *circle system*. One limb of the circle travels from the machine to the anesthesia mask, where the patient inhales it. The other limb, carrying exhaled gas, travels from the mask back to the machine, where excess carbon dioxide from the patient is filtered out. The filtered gas is mixed with fresh gas and travels back to the patient.

The same gases, minus the carbon dioxide, keep going round and round. The system is airtight, except for a pop-off valve that relieves excess pressure.

Otto was a large man with a thickly muscled neck, but by extending his head I could keep his airway clear, allowing him to continue breathing while the urologist worked. Instead of using an anesthesia mask to deliver my mix of gases, I could have assured Otto's airway by using an endotracheal tube. This is a long breathing tube (about a centimeter in diameter) inserted through the mouth all the way into the trachea.

But getting an endotracheal tube in isn't always easy, and it's usually not necessary during a cystoscopy. Most often an anesthesia mask will do.

One side effect of anesthesia is the loss of normal muscle tone. This happened to Otto. A few minutes into the case, his flaccid tongue fell back in his throat. His diaphragm continued to contract, but air couldn't get through to the lungs —his airway was obstructed. Otto was, of course, completely unconscious at this point.

Everyone loses some muscle tone during sleep—this is the cause of snoring, and of the more serious condition of sleep apnea. But the loss of tone is even greater under anesthesia, and the anesthetized patient cannot rouse herself to find a better breathing position.

I managed the problem by putting a short plastic tube called an *airway* into Otto's mouth. The airway depressed the tongue and cleared a passage for air. It wasn't as good as an endotracheal tube, which would have extended all the way into Otto's trachea, but it seemed to do the trick.

For the next ten minutes Otto was fine, but then he began to obstruct again. Now his whole mouth seemed to have relaxed backward to cover the breathing passage.

Fortunately, the gas delivery system incorporates an ingenious solution to the problem—a reservoir bag. The distensible rubber bag is connected directly into the circuit and fills with the circulating gasses. A gentle squeeze of the bag adds pressure to the system.

With one hand, I felt through Otto's skin for the back end of his jawbone, reached under it and pulled upward with my ring and small fingers. This maneuver lifted the fallen mouth tissue from the back of Otto's throat. With the remaining fingers and thumb of the same hand, I pushed the mask down hard on Otto's face to keep the seal airtight.

I kept my other hand on the anesthesia bag, squeezing it ever so slightly with every breath Otto took. This added just enough pressure to overcome the resistance and push air in. It's the same principle used by the CPAP (continuous positive airway pressure) machine to allow the sleep apneac to get a good night's rest.

Again I was ventilating Otto, but it was hard for me to hold the jaw in position. I asked the nurse to call my attending professor, Dr. Jerome.

"How much longer?" I asked the surgeon doing the case.

"I'll be done in no time. Ten minutes."

Easy for you to say, I thought. Ten minutes later Dr. Jerome arrived. He looked at me straining to keep air flowing into Otto's lungs.

"How much longer?" Dr. Jerome asked the surgeon.

"Ten minutes."

"It's not worth intubating him just for ten minutes," Dr. Jerome said to me. "Can you hold out?"

My arms were beginning to tire. An endotracheal tube would have been a godsend, but I took Dr. Jerome's hint.

"I think so," I said.

"Good lad," said Dr. Jerome. "Call if you need me."

Intubating Otto would have involved looking into his mouth with a laryngoscope (a deluxe metal tongue blade with a built-in light bulb) and directly visualizing Otto's vocal cords. (I'm using the word *visualize* here in its technical, medical sense: meaning *to see*.) This is called *direct laryngoscopy*.

Once the vocal cords are in view, it's possible to pass a semi-rigid plastic tube between the cords into the trachea. The breathing tube (endotracheal tube) secures an open passage for getting air into the lungs. Once the breathing tube is in place, it's not necessary to maneuver a patient's jaw to keep the airway open. The tube keeps the airway open by itself—it is the airway.

Some patients are easy to intubate. Some are hard. I suspected Otto was in the latter category.

Half an hour later the surgeon still hadn't finished. I didn't feel I had the strength to keep the pressure on Otto's jaw much longer. It seemed pointless to ask the surgeon how much more time he needed. I sent for Dr. Jerome.

When he came, my arms were shaking with fatigue. Otto's airway was barely open now. I stepped aside as Dr. Jerome took over to give me a rest. As his hand encircled the mask, he didn't like what he felt.

He said, "You're hard pressed to bump 'em off in cysto, but I suppose it can be done."

What Dr. Jerome meant was that losing a relatively healthy patient during a minor urology procedure was a rare mishap, but one we were nearly on the verge of. He wasn't kidding.

By this time I had a very good feel for Otto's anatomy,

and I was sure that intubating him would not be easy. His neck was short and thick and his tongue large. These physical characteristics would conspire to make it difficult for me to see his vocal cords with a laryngoscope.

Difficult intubation attempts often cause bleeding at the back of the mouth. If you get the breathing tube in, the bleeding isn't dangerous. But if you don't, the blood makes everything worse. A single drop of blood on the vocal cords can cause them to snap shut, completely obstructing the airway.

We decided to avoid the intubation attempt. While the surgeon continued to work, Dr. Jerome lifted one side of Otto's jaw and I lifted the other. Our combined force was barely enough.

Finally, the surgeon finished (the initial ten-minutes-to-go estimate had been off by an hour and a half), and I turned off the anesthetic gas. Dr. Jerome and I gradually relaxed the force on the jaw. Otto's muscle tone returned. Now that he was almost awake, he could support his own airway.

I was of two minds when, exhausted and relieved, I left Otto in the recovery room.

On the one hand, I knew his difficult airway was a product of his unusual anatomy. It was nobody's fault. I hadn't made an error in judgment. I had done the best I could, which is to say I had muddled through with the help of Dr. Jerome. All's well that ends well.

On the other hand, what would I have done without Dr. Jerome? I had pretty much run out of options and wasn't sure how I'd manage Otto's airway if I ever encountered him again as a patient. The words "hard-pressed to bump 'em off in cysto" hung darkly in my mind.

Prior to encountering Otto, I'd been pretty confident that I was mastering the techniques of anesthesiology. And I'd also been confident that those techniques, which had evolved over millions of anesthetics, were all I needed to keep anesthetized patients safe.

Now I wasn't quite so sure.

I had a thought that was new to me. Perhaps there was an inherent risk to doing anesthesia that simply came with the territory. Perhaps the risk could not be managed away even in the best of hands. Perhaps you could do everything right and still lose a patient. This was the lesson in humility that Otto taught.

The next day the surgeon called.

He said, "What did you do to my patient? His jaw is killing him, and he says he's not ever going to have surgery again if he can help it."

Dr. Jerome explained to the surgeon what had happened, and the surgeon explained to Otto, counseling him to let any future anesthesiologist know about the incident.

Otto left the hospital in disgust. Other than prescribing painkillers, there was nothing to be done. The sore jaw persisted a week (as did my sore arms.) I don't know whether Otto made good on his threat to avoid surgery, but it didn't seem a bad idea to me.

At the time of this incident, it had been a century and a third since Dr. Morton's first public anesthetic. Morton had used a clever glass vaporizer to anesthetize his patient, who breathed spontaneously through the operation. When I reflected on my experience, what I had just gone through didn't appear to be much of an advance in technique. The method I had used now seemed crude to me, and I felt in over my head.

Morton, I reckoned, had been lucky that Otto hadn't been his patient.

Two

First Do No Harm

THE MODERN ERA of surgery—indeed, of medicine—may be said to have arrived precisely at 10:15 in the morning on Friday, October 16, 1846, with Morton's public demonstration of ether anesthesia. The operation took place in the surgical theater of Massachusetts General Hospital, recognized from that time forward as the Ether Dome. Operating rooms were actual amphitheaters in those days, with rounded tiers of seating for medical students, rising away from a central stage.

Ether, "sweet vitriol," is a liquid at room temperature. It boils at 94 degrees Fahrenheit, turning easily to gas. A potent bronchodilator, it had been used for hundreds of years to treat respiratory ailments.

Many physicians and scientists had studied ether, including Sir Isaac Newton, who set it aside as an uninteresting compound. By the nineteenth century, it was used chiefly by students for ether frolics. A quantity of ether was passed among the guests at such events, who became pleasantly drunk by inhaling the vapor.

Crawford Long, a Georgia physician attending a frolic, noticed that a person injured under ether's influence didn't feel pain. Long had a brilliant idea. Wondering if ether might relieve the ordeal of surgery, he saturated a towel with it and had a patient breathe the fumes. Long then painlessly removed two small tumors from the patient's neck. After much thought, he set his fee for the case at $2.00.

Long performed his miracle in 1842, four years before Morton's demonstration. An isolated country doctor with a small practice, he didn't publish his findings. Nobody heard about it.

But surgical anesthesia was in the air, so to speak. Morton, an ambitious dentist with no university degree, had heard about ether from the physician and chemist Charles T. Jackson and began using it in his dental practice. The "new and valuable discovery" was reported in a Boston paper and Morton got himself invited to make a public demonstration. The patient, a twenty-year-old man named Edward Abbott, had a vascular lesion on the side of his neck needing removal.

Morton arrived late to the Ether Dome the day of his appointment with history—the instrument maker had only just finished the glass inhaler Morton had designed. The eminent surgeon, Dr. John Warren, irritated by Morton's delay, was about to start the procedure without him.

"Sir, your patient is ready!" scolded Warren.

Morton apologized and set to work, and Abbott was soon asleep.

"Sir, your patient is ready," said Morton, echoing Warren.

Warren took ten minutes to remove the lesion. When he was done he turned to the audience and famously pronounced, "Gentlemen, this is no humbug."

A year previously, Morton's partner, Horace Wells, had conducted a similar demonstration at Massachusetts General using laughing gas (nitrous oxide), an anesthetic less potent than ether. Wells's display had ended in failure and ridicule when the patient complained of pain.

A month after Morton's successful presentation, Dr. Oliver Wendell Holmes wrote to him proposing the term *anesthesia* (Greek for "without pain") for the magic that had been worked. A raft of new words followed. *Anesthetist* came to mean anyone who gave an *anesthetic*. A physician anesthetist such as myself, whose medical specialty is called *anesthesiology*, is known as an *anesthesiologist*.

Morton tried to disguise the nature of his anesthetic, giving it the name *Letheon*, but soon got into a bitter public struggle with Long, Jackson, and Wells to claim credit for the breakthrough. Morton tried unsuccessfully to patent ether. He died a pauper in 1868 and is buried in that loveliest of cemeteries, Mount Auburn, in Cambridge. The inscription on his headstone reads:

> *By whom, pain in surgery was averted and annulled*
> *Before whom, in all time, Surgery was Agony*
> *Since whom, science has control over pain*

Rest in peace.

     ❧ ❧ ❧

Recently, the venerable New England Journal of Medicine marked its 200th anniversary by naming the most important article in its history. The article chosen was H. J. Bigelow's 1846 report on the discovery of ether anesthesia. Bigelow was a professor of surgery at Harvard. It had been he who arranged Morton's public demonstration in the Ether Dome.

Bigelow's review gave an account of Morton's method: "A small two-necked glass globe contains the prepared vapor, together with sponges to enlarge the evaporating surface. One aperture admits the air to the interior of the globe, whence, charged with vapor, it is drawn through the second into the lungs. The inspired air thus passes through the bottle, but the expiration is diverted [out of the inhaler] by a valve in the mouth piece...."

Morton's inhaler was a vaporizer, anesthesia machine, and gas delivery system all rolled into one.

In his article, Bigelow enumerated the many failed anesthetic attempts prior to Morton and documented his own anesthesia experiments. His descriptions made two things clear. First, a revolution was brewing. Second, everyone was winging it, in over their heads, making things up as they went along.

Here is Bigelow on one of his own ether attempts gone awry:

> I found the pulse suddenly diminishing in force, so much so, that I suggested the propriety of desisting. . . .The respiration was very slow, the hands cold, and the patient insensible. Attention was now of course directed to the return of respiration and circulation. Cold allusions, as directed for poisoning with alcohol, were applied to the head, the ears were syringed, and ammonia presented to the nostrils and administered internally. For fifteen minutes the symptoms remained stationary, when it was proposed to use active exercise, as in a case of narcotism from opium. Being lifted to his feet, the patient soon made an effort to move his limbs, and the pulse became

more full, but again decreased in the sitting posture, and it was only after being compelled to walk during half an hour that the patient was able to lift his head.

Let's review the tools Bigelow had in his arsenal to treat an anesthetic overdose:

- Withdrawal of the anesthetic gas
- Cold compresses to the head
- A squirt gun aimed at the ears
- Ammonia
- Exercise

The good news was that this left a lot of room for improvement.

Ether's effects are self-limiting, making it a fortunate choice for the first anesthetic agent. Initially it stimulates both respiration and blood flow. In deeper stages of ether anesthesia, ether depresses both the heart and breathing. *But it depresses breathing more.* This means that a patient will stop inhaling ether before a heart-killing dose can be administered —exactly what was happening to Bigelow's patient.

It wasn't Bigelow's armory of techniques that saved the moment. It was the ether itself.

As excitement about anesthesia spread, new agents, some more dangerous than ether, were tried. And thus it wasn't long after the discovery of modern anesthesia that people began to die of it.

On January 28, 1848, Hannah Greener, a healthy fifteen-year-old girl from a town near Newcastle, Great Britain, underwent the removal of an ingrown toenail, for which she was given the new anesthetic, chloroform. The anesthetist, Dr. Meggison, gave this account:

> I seated her in a chair, and put a teaspoon of chloroform into a tablecloth, and held it to her nose. I told her to draw her breath naturally, which she did…. When the incision was made, she gave a struggle or jerk, which I thought was from the chloroform not having taken sufficient effect. Her eyes were closed, and I opened them, and they remained open. Her mouth was open, and her lips and face blanched. When I opened her eyes, they were congested. I called for water when I saw her face blanched, and I dashed some of it in her face. It had no effect. I then gave her some brandy, a little of which she swallowed with difficulty. I then laid her on the floor and attempted to bleed her in the arm and jugular vein. She was dead…. The time would not have been more than 3 min from her first inhaling the chloroform till her death.

For the record, Dr. Meggison's arsenal included:

- Forcing the eyes open
- Water in the face
- Brandy
- Bleeding

Though it wasn't known at the time of Hannah Greener's death, chloroform has a toxic effect on the heart. Every so often, long before it slows breathing, chloroform provokes a cardiac arrest. Ultimately, this lethal side effect caused it to be abandoned as an anesthetic.

It's apparent from Dr. Meggison's testimony he had no idea what had gone wrong with his patient.

æ æ æ

Modern anesthetic gases are derived from ether. It's still correct to say that we etherize patients, although an anesthetic begins differently now.

In the 1930s intravenous agents that produced an immediate state of unconsciousness were synthesized. The new drugs, ultra-short-acting hypnotics such as Sodium Pentothal, traveled quickly through the bloodstream to the brain.

Before then, patients had to breathe anesthesia gas to get

to sleep, which could be scary and sometimes provoked coughing fits. Intravenous induction soon replaced direct inhalation of vapor as the method of choice for starting an anesthetic.

Pentothal was still the standard when I was a resident (propofol hadn't been invented yet) and for my first year in the operating room an attending physician always stood by when I gave it. The danger is that as soon as it interrupts consciousness, Pentothal (as does propofol) also causes spontaneous respiration to stop. It does this by inhibiting the brain's respiratory center. During normal sleep, the respiratory center reminds the muscles of respiration to keep working, which is a very good thing. But under the influence of the induction agents, the respiratory center temporarily "forgets" to do this—Ondine's curse.

"Anyone can push a plunger," my attending physicians would say to me. Meaning, *what's the plan after the Pentothal goes in and the body forgets to breathe?*

I often felt, pushing that plunger then, the presence of something vast, terrifying, and doubtful nearby. I imagined being the pilot of a small boat going over the edge of a very high waterfall, a waterfall at the end of the world. The drop was one long, sickening, slow-motion glissando down to the rocks and spray below, and there was no stopping once it began. I felt that nauseating drop all through the first year of residency as I slowly gained confidence around an airway.

Then in the second year, when I was left alone to do unsupervised inductions, I felt it all over again. I felt it once more when I started in private practice many years ago.

I still feel it occasionally—much more than I'd like—now.

THREE

A HOLE IN THE NECK

THREE YEARS AFTER my encounter with Otto, I met another patient who increased my store of humility, only this time I was in private practice without a teacher to bail me out.

The patient was a forty-four-year-old woman—let's call her Rose—who needed surgery on her bladder. The procedure was more complicated than Otto's.

The urologist said he might need me to control Rose's respirations intermittently during the case, that is, to breathe for her. This can be done by squeezing the anesthesia reservoir bag, which blows air into the lungs. While it's possible to do this with an anesthesia mask strapped on the patient's face, it's easier and safer with a breathing tube in the trachea.

My plan was to put a breathing tube in Rose.

After giving Pentothal, I put a mask on Rose and squeezed the anesthesia bag. Her chest rose and fell,

21

confirming air was passing in and out of her lungs. Then I gave Rose a paralytic agent to relax the muscles around her airway.

Anesthesiologists commonly use paralytic agents (also called *muscle relaxants*) during intubation to make it easier to visualize the vocal cords. When all goes well, once the cords are visible, a breathing tube can be passed between them into the trachea.

I inserted a laryngoscope into Rose's mouth and looked for her vocal cords. No go. She had a short neck and her trachea was positioned very far forward. It was too great an angle to see around with my laryngoscope blade.

I tried another blade with a different shape. I still couldn't see Rose's vocal cords. I went back to ventilating her by mask.

Soon, the muscle relaxant (which had also paralyzed Rose's diaphragm) wore off, and Rose was breathing for herself again.

I had not done what I'd set out to do. But I had a stable, anesthetized patient who was breathing on her own.

"It's all right," the surgeon told me. "You can do the case with a mask. I won't be long."

Hadn't I heard that before?

Surgeons are notoriously bad at estimating their time. And what do they know about the difficulties of masking a patient? *Nada.*

I should have remembered Otto. I should have thought more about the two intubation attempts I had just made and the possibility that Rose now had blood in her airway. I should have woken her then and there and cancelled the case.

Knowing we were facing a difficult airway, we could have come back another day with a better, safer strategy.

One such plan would have been an awake nasal intubation—passing a small endotracheal tube through the nose and into the trachea of a conscious, spontaneously breathing patient. Sedation and local anesthesia make the technique tolerable for the owner of the nose.

Unfortunately, I didn't consider any of that.

Instead, I agreed, accepting the surgeon's glib judgment that a mask would do, and that he would be quick. I took off into the fog.

Rose wasn't as heavy as Otto, or was her neck as thick, but she became partially obstructed anyway about a half hour into the case. It's possible that her throat had become swollen from my two intubation attempts. Or perhaps I had caused some bleeding that was now irritating her vocal cords, which were partially closing in response. In any case, none of my tricks to keep the airway clear were working. No extra pair of hands materialized to help.

This time I *knew* I couldn't get a breathing tube in, because I had already tried to and failed. The urologist was only halfway through his procedure, and he wasn't having an easy time of it either.

"How's it going up there," he said.

"She's hard to ventilate."

"I need you to paralyze her and control her respirations," he said.

"I thought you told me you weren't going to need that," I said.

"Five minutes. That's all I need."

Paralyzing her again now, however, was out of the question. The one thing I had going in my favor was that Rose was still breathing for herself. At this point I didn't want to interfere with that.

I remembered Otto, and a panicky feeling began building. If I lost the airway I would lose Rose, and I might lose the airway at any time. I sent a message to the front desk asking for backup. No other anesthesiologist was available.

The urologist, intent on his procedure, was of no help. My mind began to wander. Oh, to be a resident again, when plenty of help was always around. Why were airways so troublesome? So complicated? Why not easy and simple? Why couldn't every patient just be born with a hole in the neck leading straight to the trachea?

Deep in my brain, something clicked.

"She needs a tracheotomy," I said.

"Whatever you think," said the surgeon. "I just need you to paralyze her."

A tracheotomy involves making an incision in the front of the neck and creating a direct opening into the trachea, through which a short breathing tube is passed. Was it overkill? Perhaps. But overkill was better than kill.

A head and neck surgeon, Dr. Anthony, had just finished a case and was still in the hospital. We summoned him to the room.

Anthony and I worked well together. I'd learned by then to stay on good terms with all head and neck surgeons. They have an intimate knowledge of airway anatomy and understand better than any other surgical specialists the difficulties anesthesiologists face.

By now Rose had respiratory stridor, a croupy sound caused by air turbulence, and a signal to everyone in the room that all wasn't well at the head of the table.

The pulse oximeter read 92 percent. The number meant that Rose was still getting enough oxygen, but it was barely reassuring. Five minutes before, the number had been 94 percent. As with Otto, I might have muddled through to the end of the case, but I was done with muddling. The surgeon still needed muscle relaxation, and it wasn't safe to provide that relaxation until Rose's airway was secure.

Dr. Anthony agreed.

The circulating nurse hastily prepped Rose's neck and got an emergency tracheotomy tray. The urologist abandoned his procedure for the moment to assist Anthony. The two men worked in close quarters for ten minutes while I struggled to keep the airway open.

Emergency is not a word you like to see paired with *tracheotomy*. The neck brims with a profuse tangle of blood vessels lying in ambush for the unwary surgeon. If you lose control of the operative field during a tracheotomy—meaning if the bleeding becomes uncontrollable—you've just run out of options.

After an eternity Anthony called out, "Trach tube!"

The scrub nurse passed the tube to Anthony, who slid it into the trachea. The ordeal was over. I connected my breathing circuit to that blessed tube, a direct path to Rose's lungs.

It was safe to paralyze Rose now with a muscle relaxant, which the urologist required to finish his case. Rose ended up with a neck scar she hadn't bargained for, but she'd live to tell her grandchildren about it. I had egg on my face and some explaining to do, but it beat the alternative.

A week later I sat with Rose and we talked. She was philosophical, which was more than I felt I deserved.

"I made an error in judgment. I should have cancelled the case when I couldn't intubate you," I said to her.

"You kept me alive," she said. "You were wonderful."

I hadn't been wonderful.

What I had been was lucky that the right man was around when we needed him.

FOUR

HOW TO STOP BREATHING

HOW DO PEOPLE breathe, and what stops them?

Well, people breathe because they do. If you like simple explanations, read no further, because the control of breathing is fiendishly complex.

The heart of the system is a group of pacemaker cells in the respiratory center of the brain's medulla. The pacemaker cells rhythmically stimulate motor neurons controlling the diaphragm—the primary breathing muscle. Contraction of the diaphragm stretches out the lungs and causes inhalation; its relaxation causes exhalation.

The pacemaker cells continue to rhythmically stimulate the diaphragm rain or shine, all day and all night. It takes a massive anesthetic overdose to shut them down.

A basic meditation technique is to follow one's breath, that is, to let breathing occur without trying to influence it.

Essentially, this means observing the respiratory center operating on its own. The meditator has a direct experience of an intelligence at work not governed by conscious thought.

The respiratory center is subject to influence from above and below. To demonstrate respiratory influence from above, kindly have your frontal cortex send a message to your medulla to stop breathing. Go ahead and do it now, it's perfectly safe—I'm a doctor. You'll stop breathing for a while, but eventually your pacemaker cells will override your will, and you'll find yourself breathing again.

You are more than your conscious will.

What happened? Influence from below. There are sensors everywhere in the body that send information about your respiratory needs back to the respiratory center—sensors in the brain and blood vessels, sensors in the lungs, sensors in muscles and joints, sensors in your nose.

Don't believe me about the nose? What do you think a sneeze is?

It turns out that the primary signal causing the respiratory center to cause you to breathe is not a lack of oxygen. It's a buildup of carbon dioxide in your blood. Carbon dioxide, you may remember from biology, is a by-product of the burning of sugar deep in the body's cells. And it's the burning of sugar that gives you energy to go on living and breathing.

It's said that the Greek philosopher Diogenes—the guy who carried a lamp around looking for an honest man—

committed suicide by holding his breath. I don't believe it. Long before death, he would have lost consciousness, and the pacemaker cells in his respiratory center would have kicked in again.

I often tell my son Nick, who is ten, to listen to his body, such as by resting when he's sick. Our conversations go like this:

Me: "Your body will tell you when it's time to go out and play."

Nick: "My brain tells me."

Me: "Your body is the boss."

Nick: "My brain is the boss."

Me: "Want to bet?"

Nick: "Yeah."

Me: "Have your brain tell your body to stop breathing."

Here Nick makes a show of holding his breath, but sneaks in a few when he thinks I'm not looking.

Nick: "See—my brain is stronger. I didn't breathe."

Me: "You're breathing now. You have to breathe to talk."

Nick: "Not me."

So great is the illusion of conscious control.

༈ ༈ ༈

Turning off the respiratory center (anesthetics such as Pentothal do this temporarily) is one way to stop breathing. There are two others: muscle paralysis and restriction or obstruction of the airway.

The modern history of muscle paralysis begins with curare, which was discovered by the indigenous peoples of tropical rain forests. These early chemists refined the sap of certain vines into a toxin into which they dipped their blow darts.

Specimens of curare plant arrived in Europe in the eighteenth century, though the drug remained only a laboratory tool until 1940. At that time psychiatrists began using it to blunt the fracture-causing seizures that frequently resulted from electroshock therapy. Curare was introduced into anesthesia practice in 1942.

Curare works by stopping nervous transmission at the junction of nerve and muscle cell. The brain issues a command; the electric impulse travels normally down the appropriate nerve, but stops where the nerve connects to muscle. The muscle doesn't get the message to contract.

Curare affects voluntary muscle cells only—the diaphragm, muscles of the arms, legs, head, neck, and body trunk. It doesn't directly impact the heart.

For anesthesiologists, curare was a boon. Prior to its use, it was only possible to relax abdominal muscles in surgery by using near-toxic levels of anesthesia gas. With curare, the dose of gas could be lowered. Anesthesia immediately became less dangerous.

In addition, although breathing tubes had been invented long before commercial curare became available, the process of passing one through the mouth and into the trachea had always proved a struggle, reserved for a few experts. An awkward attempt at intubation might cause the vocal cords to snap shut (laryngospasm), creating a medical emergency.

With curare, and the newer paralytic agents that followed, the vocal cords relax into an open position. Moreover, with relaxation of the muscles of the head and neck, inserting the laryngoscope becomes less of a struggle. Visualizing the vocal cords and slipping a tube through them gets easier.

Of course, there's a cost to using muscle relaxants: they stop patients from breathing—Ondine's curse again. The brain issues the command, but the diaphragm doesn't hear it.

I had used a powerful, short-acting relaxant called Anectine on Rose. But even with the profound muscle relaxation that accompanied it, my attempts to intubate her failed owing to her peculiar anatomy. Rose's vocal cords were beyond the reach of my laryngoscope.

ò& ò& ò&

The third way that breathing stops, obstruction or restriction of the airway, is a problem of anatomy. Anatomy is what you need to know to find your way to the vocal cords and, when necessary, to get a breathing tube through them.

The body's three-dimensional structure is so complex that it took many centuries for doctors to unravel its mysteries. Any first-year medical student can verify the difficulties of envisioning and memorizing that structure. In my day there were no scanners or computer graphics to ease this prodigious cerebral effort. What we had was a book of drawings to look at and a cadaver to dissect.

In my medical school, four students, two on a side, were assigned to each cadaver in first-year anatomy lab. I still remember the names of my partners: Skip, Larry, and Jon. We jokingly called our cadaver Walt, because Walt Disney had recently died and willed his body to science.

Anatomy was no joke, however. It was a problem in spatial relations harder than any academic subject I've encountered before or since. Anatomy lab was also a kind of baptism. Most of us had never seen a dead person before, much less cut one open.

A sign in a corner of the lab proclaimed in Latin: *Here the dead instruct for the benefit of the living.* The four of us slaved over Walt, gently and not so gently teasing apart his

32

intricate structure for nine godawful months.

"My grandmother told me Walt wasn't a real body," Skip announced to the rest of us one day. "She says it must be a plastic model because they wouldn't give us a real body."

This took a moment to sink in.

"Pretty good model," said Jon.

Plastic models didn't come soaked in formaldehyde, as far as I knew, but the idea provided comic relief for the day.

"Well, why not?" said Larry. "I mean, if they can send a man to the moon…"

By the end of that year I had accomplished one of the supreme intellectual acts of my life. I had a mental picture of every one of the hundreds of bones, muscles, tendons, nerves, blood vessels, lymphatics, glands, and organs that comprised a human being. The picture encapsulated a billion years of evolution, and was dazzling in scope, miraculous in detail, incomparably beautiful.

A year later I had forgotten most of it. I forgot it because I had no use for it, as if I had memorized a train schedule without ever taking a train. To hold anatomy in your head, it needs to count, and it was only after meeting patients like Otto and Rose that anatomy really began to count for me.

Today I hold in my heart the precise anatomy of air and breathing. I've kept it there ever since my anesthesia residency. To me it's bread and butter, alpha and omega, life and death. I think about it constantly. It's more than a picture, it's a living, three-dimensional movie, and the movie loops day in and day out in my mind.

The movie goes like this:

Close-up on a molecule of oxygen gas, two oxygen atoms tethered in perfect harmony. The molecule floats randomly about the universe. Eons pass.

Dissolve to a bright summer's day in Ireland. Laughter. A young man and woman at a picnic.

He takes her in his muscular arms and pulls her close. She knows he is about to kiss her and instinctively draws in a breath as she closes her eyes.

Her diaphragm contracts downward to enlarge the chest cavity, stretching her spongy lung tissue like a drawn-out accordion, dropping the pressure inside the tiny air sacs that populate her lungs.

Summer air flows in, the taste of July in her mouth. The molecule of oxygen, just passing by, is drawn upward and then straight back through her nasal passages, joining thousands, millions, billions of other molecules now flying the same route. If her mouth happens to be open, as it is now, a parallel stream of molecules passes through her lips, over her tongue, under her palate, and between her tonsils.

The streams traveling horizontally through her mouth and nose meet at the back of her throat where they run smack into a vertical wall of tissue. Abruptly they change direction by ninety degrees and plunge downward, the flow of air taking a right-angled path.

Deep in her neck the pathway forks into a back tunnel leading to the stomach and a forward passage to the lungs.

Bypassing the rear tunnel, the stream of air rushes forward and encounters her vocal cords—two thin membranes of tissue that meet in the center like a curtain. Just now the curtain has opened into a V shape, and air flows through the V into the trachea. From there it follows the sinuous, ever-narrowing course of the bronchial tree through the lungs until at last it reaches a microscopic air sac, where molecular oxygen can pass through a cellular membrane into her bloodstream.

The couple kiss. She holds her breath, then lets it out. Her heart is going like mad. Yes. Yes, she will. Yes.

          ❧ ❧ ❧

Anesthesiologists, you will know by now, make a big fuss about breathing. Specifically, they fuss over the problem of getting that molecule of oxygen from under the nose to an air sac in the lung when the patient is not doing it on her own.

As it happens when the respiratory center takes a break.

Or when muscle relaxants prevent the diaphragm from contracting.

Or when any part of the airway is restricted or obstructed or collapses on itself.

The last being what happened to Otto and Rose.

An obstructed airway, it turns out, has proved to be a much thornier problem than a switched-off respiratory center or a paralyzed diaphragm. The reason is simple enough. An active respiratory center isn't necessary to ensure that a supply of oxygen gets to the lungs. Nor is a functioning diaphragm. But there does need to be an airway.

If you're in the anesthesia trade, as long as you have an airway you can ventilate a patient. You can wait for a switched-off respiratory center to turn itself back on, which is what almost always happens. You can also wait for a muscle relaxant to wear off (or be reversed by an antidote) and the diaphragm to kick in.

But you can't wait for an obstructed airway to right itself. You've got to right it. You must find a way to ventilate your patient because when oxygen stops getting to the lungs, brain cells start to die in about four minutes.

That's the airway time frame: four minutes.

Doctors have been mulling over the airway problem for a long time. Why such a complex airway? Why the hard-to-see-around, right-angled path of air? Why a windpipe so far from the mouth and nose? Why a larynx so dangerously close to the path food must take?

The human larynx is situated higher in the necks of infants than adults. Its drop into adult position is part of normal human development. At one time the falling larynx was thought unique to our species, and enabling of speech. But this theory was an oversimplification. A descending larynx has since been observed in other, non-talking animals.

Subtle is the Lord. We don't know the reasons for the downward wandering larynx. What we do know is that the circuitous, hard-to-visualize, right-angled path of air is the one we're stuck with.

FIVE

LOSING THE WAR

I ONCE READ an essay titled "Losing the War" whose relevance will become apparent shortly. The author, Lee Sandlin, was writing about the psychology of war. The essay appeared in the *Chicago Reader* in March 1997.

In his essay, Sandlin proposed that the mindset of war could be best explained by two Viking terms. The first term was *berserker*, familiar to me as a man in battle who killed without restraint.

The second Viking term was *fey*, and this was new to me. Here is what Sandler wrote:

> People now understand [fey] to mean effeminate. Previously it meant odd, and before that uncanny, fairylike. That was back when fairyland was the most sinister place people could imagine. The Old Norse word meant "doomed." It was used

to refer to an eerie mood that would come over people in battle, a kind of transcendent despair.... Sometimes men say afterward that the most terrifying moment of any battle is seeing a fey look on the faces of the soldiers standing next to them.

I've never been in combat. When I read those words I had no feeling for what fey meant in a practical sense. It seemed to have nothing to do with me, as my life was far removed from a battlefield. But that was before the day I met Sam, with whose airway I fought a losing battle.

This is what happened:

Sam was to undergo a minor urology procedure. (What is it about urology procedures and airways? I don't know.)

Sam was a cheerful, healthy man of forty-six. I performed my usual pre-operative physical exam. Although Sam was heavyset, nothing during my exam warned of a difficult airway. I planned to do the case with a mask, allowing Sam to breathe spontaneously.

After I gave Pentothal, Sam stopped breathing. This was a normal and temporary side effect of the drug—the respiratory center on hold.

I put an airway in Sam's mouth and positioned the anesthesia mask over his face, pressing the mask down to seal it against the skin. I squeezed the bag to push some air into

Sam's lungs, my usual procedure.

Nothing happened.

I repositioned the mask and tried again, hooking one finger around the angle of Sam's jaw and lifting to clear the airway. Still, no oxygen got to his lungs.

Then I did something inexplicable.

Instead of waiting for breathing to start up on its own (which it always does), I felt the soft tissue in Sam's neck and decided he'd be easy to intubate. I gave him the standard paralytic agent, Anectine, to relax his airway muscles and facilitate intubation.

I inserted my laryngoscope. To my surprise, I couldn't find the vocal cords. The right angle of Sam's airway was too severe. I couldn't see around it.

I shoved the tube in anyway, hoping it would find its way by blind luck. But it was obvious when I tried to ventilate through it that the tube was in the esophagus.

Agitated now, I pulled the tube out and reapplied the mask. I still couldn't ventilate Sam by mask. Neither could I intubate him. And he was now completely paralyzed.

Sam's respiratory center by now had started up again and was signaling his diaphragm to breathe. But the Anectine was blocking the message from getting through.

Can't intubate, can't ventilate, paralyzed patient—the most dire airway emergency.

The oxygen saturation started to fall. Besides displaying

the saturation on a monitor, pulse oximeters emit a short tone coincident with every heart beat. If the saturation is high, the tone pitch is high. If the saturation falls, the tone falls in pitch.

The effect of hearing a beat-by-beat drop in pitch is alarming, and it's intended to be. The room now filled with a series of falling tones, the sound of Sam's blood turning blue.

"What can I do?" said the nurse.

"Get help," I said.

My insides turned buttery as I began to grasp the magnitude of my error. It was cardinal and unforgivable: I had paralyzed a patient whom I couldn't mask. It was something I'd been taught not to do, and I'd never done before or since.

To this day, I can't say precisely what provoked this lapse. But *lapse* is too kind a word. Hubris, the Greeks might have called it. Delirium is more like it.

Had there been time to call a surgeon to do a tracheotomy, I would have considered it. But there was no time. I had four minutes before Sam's brain cells would start to die. I'd already used up two of them.

One available instrument might have helped, a flexible fiberoptic laryngoscope. This was a long, thin tube through which light could bend and around which an endotracheal tube could slide.

With fiberoptics, reluctant vocal cords could sometimes be coaxed into view. But the fiberoptic laryngoscope was a new device, extremely difficult to use, and I wasn't familiar enough with it.

I've since learned to use the fiberoptic scope, and other similar airway tools that were about to come into existence. But face masks, ordinary laryngoscopes, and tracheotomies were pretty much the whole show then. Hardly an arsenal, you'd think, to justify overconfidence.

Except in a fool.

The pitch of the pulse oximeter continued its dismaying fall. The saturation was now 60 percent. I continued trying to force air into Sam's lungs without success.

The room was a blur. The nurses probably continued to ask me questions and I might have answered, but I don't remember.

I groped for an idea, but none came, other than the idle thought that maybe the Anectine, which generally lasts five to ten minutes, would wear off before it was too late. But Sam still couldn't breathe. He would die and I would be the cause.

I looked at the saturation. It was 40 percent. I had never seen it that low. Sam's blood was mostly empty of oxygen. But you didn't need an oximeter to know that. Sam was blue now.

The ship was going to the bottom.

Then a strange thing happened. Something in my soul gave. I felt my heart slow and my head clear. The panic subsided, along with the desire to do anything at all.

I watched Sam's cyanotic body, the color of a moonlit sea, without alarm. There was nothing to be done. Sam would die. That was all right.

None of this was a conscious decision on my part. I wasn't trying to rationalize. It happened in my body. My body surrendered. It was a great relief. I was at peace.

You might say it was the final humility.

I had never felt this way before or since. The experience was singular. As I read what I've written, it seems terrible to me now—a breach of the Hippocratic oath, a denial of everything I hold sacred. How could I abandon my patient? How could I stop caring and stop trying?

I can't tell you how. I can only tell you that there was no defense against it.

I understand now that what I was feeling was fey. And I also understand why the most terrifying thing in battle is to see a fey look on the soldier next to you. It's total surrender to the unbearable.

Fey is probably what happens to captains who go down with their ships. Lee Sandlin, whose essay I quoted from previously, thinks it happens to whole nations on the brink of losing a war.

In the middle of that eerie doom the door of the room burst open. I watched serenely as Rob Tavers, an anesthesiologist who had been working down the hall, ran in. Tavers was a huge man, six feet six inches tall, with enormous and powerful hands. He took the mask from me and held it down over Sam's face with both thumbs and index fingers, simultaneously lifting both sides of Sam's jaw with his middle and ring fingers. Then he set his chin on the top of the mask and rested all his weight on it.

"Take the bag," he said.

The resistance was so great that when I first squeezed the bag, it detached from its connector and shot to the floor. I picked it up and twisted it violently back on. Then I squeezed again using both hands.

We were improvising. That is to say, Tavers was improvising and dragging me along. What we were doing later came to be called *two-man ventilation*. It was a version of what Dr. Jerome and I did with Otto's airway years before, the principle being that four trained hands working in concert were better than two.

I looked at Sam's chest. Did it go up and down? Maybe some oxygen was getting in. Tavers and I persisted. Half a minute later the tones of the pulse oximeter slowly began to rise.

A tiny stream of oxygen was getting through.

A few more minutes and Sam began to make feeble respiratory attempts. The Anectine was finally wearing off. The intense blue of his skin softened to violet.

Tavers stayed ten minutes. When he left I took over holding the mask. I didn't need to squeeze the bag as Sam was breathing now. He was waking up.

The oxygen saturation rose to 60 percent, then 70

percent, then, suddenly, 90 percent. The surgeon and I agreed to cancel the case, a good thing as I was in no shape to continue. We took Sam to the recovery room.

A half hour later, impossibly, Sam was sitting up in bed and talking.

I was still a basket case, but Sam had all his faculties. All his muscles worked. No harm, but a very big foul.

"Take the rest of the day off," Tavers said to me.

I spent an hour with Sam, explaining everything. Later I wrote a letter, telling him to give it to the anesthesiologist if he ever needed surgery again.

Sam needed no telling. He had woken up with a feeling that he couldn't breathe. The Anectine had outlasted the Pentothal by a couple of minutes.

I probably could have obliterated the memory of his paralysis had I the presence of mind to give Sam a sedative once Tavers and I were in control of his airway. But my mind was only beginning to emerge from fey when Sam started to recover.

Sam was understanding about it.

"I could feel air stretching my lungs," he said. "I just didn't like the feeling."

"It must have been scary," I said.

"It was. You looked scared, too."

ঌ ঌ ঌ

Every anesthesiologist has Sam, Rose, and Otto stories, moments when events in an operating room spiral dangerously out of control. Those moments terrify because the job of anesthesia is to control everything you can think of that matters to life—heart, lung, muscle, blood, brain, metabolism, air.

If you lose control and don't get it back, the outcome is always bad. The most sickening outcome is to lose a patient.

"When you operate on people, some of them will die," a head and neck surgeon, a giant in his field, said to me once when I was an intern.

He was trying to console me after a patient of his whom I was caring for died from a surgical complication the night after an operation.

He was right, but I've noticed that anesthesiologists take death harder than most other physicians. I think this comes of the anesthesiologist's object to incapacitate his patient—to be both Ondine's instrument and antidote. A clinician wants to take his patient as far away from death as possible. An anesthesiologist must take him closer.

Whatever the reason, an intimacy develops between anesthesiologists and the defenseless, sleeping bodies they're supposed to be protecting on the night sea journey. When giving anesthesia, I can't help feeling my patients as part of myself. It makes sense to me now that I so identified with

47

Sam that fey overcame me as I watched him dying.

Shortly after the experience with Sam, I began to have a recurring nightmare. In the dream, I'm giving a patient a dose of medicine that does him irreparable harm. The monitors tell me something terrible has happened.

I know the reckoning will be severe. But I don't know what the offending medicine is—I don't know what I've done.

I wonder if Dr. Meggison had a similar nightmare about Hannah Greener, after she slipped away in that long-ago operating parlor near Newcastle.

When I'm having this dream, I'm like Dr. Meggison: I can't do anything about the situation. The feeling is unimaginably terrifying.

Then something more terrible happens in the dream: I start not to care.

Fey returns.

The nightmare has come less often over time but still visits now and then. It's a relief when I wake to find it's just been a dream. I suppose my psyche is wrestling with the words of that head and neck surgeon: *some will die*.

In my head, I know death is inevitable. The dream takes the knowledge into the body. It's both a spur and a warning: let it not be your fault. *Let fey not come again.*

After the horrific episode with Sam I determined to improve my airway skills, which I now saw as inadequate, despite my several years of practice. I began using the flexible fiberoptic laryngoscope during routine intubations. I wanted to be as comfortable with it as with a standard laryngoscope, so that I could reach for it with confidence in an emergency.

It took an extra five minutes to do each of those intubations, and surgeons complained of the delay. I let them complain.

I finally mastered the flexible fiberoptic scope, and it's enabled me to accomplish more and more difficult intubations. But it wasn't a panacea. Some airways were beyond even its reach.

In the years since I encountered Sam, new contraptions have appeared that have given the anesthesiologist a greater purchase on the difficult airway. Some are strange looking and take time to master. But so what?

This is my attitude now: a new gizmo for jousting with the right-angled path of air? Something to increase my odds?

Where do I sign?

Six

Air Control

CONTROL OF BREATHING has been central to anesthesia from the very beginning. After W. T. G. Morton's initial success with ether, it soon became apparent to physicians that spontaneous respirations through an ether inhaler left too much to chance. Had Otto been Morton's first patient, for example, the demonstration in the Ether Dome might have turned out very differently.

Easily obstructed airways weren't the only problem that needed solving. Prior to the advent of ether, surgery was of necessity rapid and restricted to accessible areas of the body such as arms and legs. After ether was discovered, surgeons gained the luxury of time. The interior of the body beckoned, and operations grew longer and more invasive.

Surgeons began devising even more daring procedures, undreamed of before ether. For many of the new operations, a safe airway needed to be guaranteed. How to keep a patient breathing, for example, while operating on her face, in her mouth, or inside her lungs?

Inhalers grew more elaborate than Morton's. Soon a rough version of the anesthesia mask was added to the anesthetist's armory, and then endotracheal (breathing) tubes.

The idea of breathing tubes was very old. Hippocrates himself had worried about the airway. The first description of endotracheal intubation is in his *Treatise on Air*, written twenty-five hundred years ago: "One should introduce a cannula into the trachea along the jawbone so that air can be drawn into the lungs."

We have no record of how Hippocrates actually put his method into practice. We do know that the first modern endotracheal intubations were blind—an anesthetist shoved a metal breathing tube down a patient's throat and hoped it would land in the trachea.

By the beginning of the twentieth century, rubber breathing tubes replaced metal ones. And the modern laryngoscope—the device for directly visualizing the vocal cords—had appeared.

Each advance in surgery coincided with an advance in anesthesia technique. The advent of lung surgery provides a striking illustration of such hand-in-hand progress.

Physicians had long known that the thoracic cavity, which houses the heart and lungs, was beyond reach of the surgeon's knife. If you tried cutting through the thoracic wall to expose the lung the results were lethal. The lung collapsed as the patient grew short of breath and died.

No one knew why.

Doctors assumed the chest wall to be one of those mysterious natural barriers that could never be breached, the same way sailors once thought that they couldn't sail around Africa, and pilots thought that they couldn't fly into clouds. Those who tried didn't live to tell about it.

We now know that an intact chest wall protects the thoracic cavity from the weight of the atmosphere. Without a sealed chest wall to protect them, the lungs would be squeezed like a sponge.

Normal breathing is controlled by the diaphragm, the muscle situated underneath the chest cavity. When the diaphragm contracts downward on inhalation, it creates a vacuum in the space around the lungs, causing the lungs to expand and air to flow in through the mouth and nose.

An incision in the chest wall short-circuits the breathing cycle. Now when the diaphragm contracts, air from the atmosphere is sucked into the chest cavity through the hole. The vacuum around the lung dissipates and the lung can't expand. No air flows in through the mouth and nose. Soon the pressure around the affected lung builds up to equal atmospheric weight, and the lung is squeezed empty of air.

By the end of the nineteenth century, anesthetists had

solved the problem of the chest cavity. Endotracheal tubes (breathing tubes such as envisioned by Hippocrates) were passed through the mouth or nose into the trachea. Connecting a breathing tube to a bellows (a primitive ventilator) made it possible to force air into the lungs mechanically. With an anesthesiologist controlling respiration this way, it was safe for the surgeon to incise the chest wall.

Anesthesia technique and equipment continued to advance throughout the twentieth century. Rubber masks and breathing tubes gave way to plastic ones. Laryngoscopes sprouted tiny light bulbs, and an array of new blade shapes grew to follow the right-angled path of air and give better direct exposure of the vocal cords.

Ventilators developed from simple bellows into complex electronic machines. A steady parade of new anesthetic agents got safer and more effective. Electronic monitoring devices such as the pulse oximeter allowed more exact measurement of a patient's clinical state.

In the last quarter of the twentieth century, two developments in particular have dramatically improved airway safety.

The first, which I mentioned in connection with Sam, is fiberoptics, the technology of bending light.

As ingenious as ordinary laryngoscopes have become, some airways remain impenetrable to them. It turns out that not all right-angled paths are alike. In some patients, the angle is less severe and the vocal cords at the end of the path are fairly easy to visualize. In other patients—Rose and Sam, for example—the turn is sharper, and the vocal cords cannot be coaxed into direct view by any laryngoscope blade. It's hard to pass a breathing tube through a pathway you cannot see.

But if a severely curved laryngoscope blade is constructed with embedded fibers that conduct light, then it becomes possible to see around an extreme airway bend. The vocal cords become visible by looking through the optical fibers.

The first fiberoptic laryngoscopes were crude and difficult to use, much as the first direct laryngoscopes were. But they got better. Today fiberoptic laryngoscopes, which come in various shapes and sizes, have a place on every anesthesiologist's cart.

One other late twentieth century airway development had an important impact on anesthesia safety. It was an improvement on the standard anesthesia mask, the kind of mask I used on Otto and Rose—and that didn't work on Sam.

You might suppose from the difficulties I've described that the standard anesthesia mask leaves something wanting in the way of airway management. After all, if it's so easy to lose control of an airway using an anesthesia mask, why not simply put a full-fledged breathing tube in every patient?

There are three reasons not to do this.

First, the stories of Otto, Rose, and Sam are unusual.

Most of the time, face masks work, at least for a while.

Second, intubation is more invasive than masking. It irritates the trachea and calls for deeper anesthesia. You like to avoid it if you don't really need it.

Finally, a severe right-angled path makes some patients (such as Otto and Rose, for example) very difficult to intubate.

Dr. Archie Brain, an aptly named British anesthesiologist with an inventive streak, is in full agreement about the problems of the anesthesia mask.

The mask had been around for the better part of a century when Dr. Brain began to think about improving it. But instead of simply tinkering, he had the idea to abandon it completely.

What if, Dr. Brain reasoned, instead of applying a mask to the face to cover the mouth and nose, he applied a smaller mask *inside* the mouth—all the way at the back of the throat —to go around the right angle and cover the larynx directly?

Such a device would obviate the problem of the tongue falling back to obstruct the airway. Rather than being a face mask, the new gadget would be a *laryngeal mask*.

A laryngeal mask wouldn't pass between the vocal cords and into the trachea, like an endotracheal tube does. Instead, it would sit on top of the larynx without going in, just as a standard mask covers the face without going in the mouth. But it would protect the larynx from a fallen tongue.

Dr. Brain began to experiment with cadavers to see

whether he could devise a shape that would work. He settled on an oblong form for his new mask—elliptical at one end, tapering to a point at the other.

He attached an inflatable cuff around the perimeter and fastened a semi-rigid plastic tube to the mask. The tube ran from the mask (which sat just above the vocal cords), around the right-angled path of air, out the mouth, and connected to the breathing circuit.

Archie Brain called the device the LMA—the laryngeal mask airway.

An LMA is easy to put in. You don't need a muscle relaxant. You insert it into the mouth of a sleeping patient and push it to the back of the throat until it dead-ends at the tracheal inlet over the vocal cords. Then you inflate the cuff.

With the LMA you don't need to see a thing. You don't need to see around the right-angled path. You put it in by feel.

The laryngeal mask provides a better path for air than a standard mask and does so consistently and reliably. The airway is better because with the LMA, it doesn't matter if the tongue and mouth tissue fall back in the throat—oxygen is traveling through the plastic tube of the LMA.

Introduced over two decades ago, the LMA became immediately popular with anesthesiologists. It's such an improvement that I rarely do a case now with a face mask. In the years since I began using the LMA, I've had only one patient I couldn't ventilate with it, and that was probably caused by my inexperience.

I still use a face mask at the beginning of every general anesthetic, but only to ventilate with pure oxygen for few moments before either intubating or putting in an LMA.

If I can't ventilate with a face mask, I immediately switch to an LMA, even if I eventually want to put in an endotracheal tube. You can count on the LMA in a way you could never count on a face mask.

The laryngeal mask has smoothed out anesthesia for thousands—maybe millions—of patients. It's also saved lives. I wish I'd had it as a resident.

An LMA wouldn't have solved Rose's airway problem—she needed to be intubated. But it would have worked for Otto and Sam and rendered their stories mundane and boring. And mundane, boring stories—not interesting ones—are the ideal in an operating room.

Seven

Zero Hour

IT'S NOW CLOSE to 6:00 a.m., and I'm driving in the dark down a mountain pass approaching the hospital, thinking about my cases for the day. I've been assigned four procedures: a femoral artery repair, two knee explorations, and a hysterectomy.

From the moment I'm assigned to a case I begin obsessing about how to proceed. I'm always thinking of the central problem and the dangers. I think about my tools. I think about the worst things that can happen. And I think about the judgments I'm going to be called on to exercise.

The devilish thing about good judgment is that it comes by way of experience, which comes by way of bad judgment. The best you can do with your mistakes of judgment is to learn from them, as I've learned from countless patients, such as Otto and Rose. And of course, Sam. They all ride in the car with me, Otto and Rose in the back seat while Sam rides shotgun.

Since you can't possibly have seen every problem in your career (or even most), much good judgment must be acquired secondhand from the medical literature. Firsthand judgment, though more painfully obtained than judgment from books and journals, is also more durable. But the truth is that more than having been prepared either by reading or experience, I'd rather be just plain lucky.

Soon after arriving at the hospital I walk into the pre-op holding room to visit my first patient. One look tells me this is not a lucky day.

Charlie, the patient to undergo the femoral artery repair, is sitting up in bed. Because he's a vascular patient, I know his femoral artery isn't the only bad artery he has. All over his body, Charlie has bad arteries: stiff, narrowed, and hardened with arteriosclerotic plaque.

Bad blood vessels never help an anesthetic, but that's the least of the trouble. Charlie is sitting up in bed because he can't breathe lying down. He looks to be 400 pounds and has a thick neck, which may signal a difficult airway. A cannula blows oxygen into his nose, which he inhales in shallow, rapid breaths. Beads of sweat gather on Charlie's forehead.

Strangely, or perhaps not so strangely, looking at Charlie makes me think of Sam. Sam always comes to mind when I sense danger. I think of Sam and I begin anticipating things.

Of course, the danger from Sam came out of left field— his airway from hell was unexpected. In Charlie's case I'm already expecting trouble, and the source of trouble is not only Charlie's potentially bad airway, it's his bad everything.

I know it's magical thinking to believe you can anticipate every problem. It's magical thinking to expect that anticipating a problem will always solve it. You can do everything right and still see things go terribly wrong. Yet what am I here for if not to anticipate the worst?

I steady my nerves. I say a brief hello to Charlie and excuse myself to find his medical chart.

The pre-operative visit is really a scouting expedition. I like to start with the chart because it's full of intriguing news —comments on previous procedures, medical histories, hospital progress notes, and test results. It's a record of everyone's experience with the patient, maps and weather reports for the night sea journey we're about to undertake.

When I talk to and examine a patient I'm comparing my own impressions to what others have said in the chart, paying particular attention to the airway. Later I'll ask the surgeon about the operating conditions she'll need. As a dutiful boatman, I need to weigh all the information against my own experience. My judgment, such as it is, is called for. The process is an unfolding one, a lot happening unconsciously before everything coalesces into a plan.

But not in Charlie's case.

With Charlie the plan is born the moment I glance his way—Athena sprung entire from the head of Zeus—and the plan never lets go.

The plan is this:

Get the biggest, fattest breathing tube I have into Charlie as soon as I can after he goes to sleep, and then ventilate the crap out of him.

Squeeze the bag with all the force and rapidity I can muster for the entire case and then forget about taking Charlie to the recovery room. Instead, take him straight to the intensive care unit after the operation is done, breathing tube in place.

This is providing I can get a breathing tube into him after he's asleep. If not, I'll do it when he's still awake.

Once in the ICU I'll call a lung specialist. I won't consider for a moment removing that breathing tube. Let the lung specialist, like Scarlett O'Hara, worry about it tomorrow. It will be one less problem—and Charlie's doctors will have many problems to worry about—for the first post-op day.

I don't often have to give an anesthetic to a patient this risky, and I don't know whether this fact increases or lessens my discomfort. Charlie is poised on a knife edge. He has me scared, because his life will depend on the plan going well. His bad arteries, his potentially difficult airway, his morbid obesity, and his impending respiratory failure—all conspire malignantly against him.

꙳ ꙳ ꙳

I circle back to Charlie's bedside and he shakes my hand. His face has an innocent, puzzled expression, making him look younger than his fifty-two years. On the shelf behind him lie blood-pressure cuffs of different sizes. The nurse has apparently had trouble finding one to fit him.

Through the window I can see the foothills I was traversing half an hour ago. It's sunup and the treetops glow orange against the stark blue air.

"Hey, doc," is all Charlie says.

He's used to doctors and bears my questions with grace. He keeps his answers brief because long answers would tax his breathing. I listen to his chest through my stethoscope and decide he'll benefit from a bronchodilator this morning, a drug to widen the air passages in his lungs. I order it to be given right away through a handheld nebulizer.

I examine Charlie's mouth and neck to get an idea how difficult it will be to get the breathing tube in. Ordinarily a patient undergoing a femoral artery repair doesn't need a breathing tube, but Charlie isn't an ordinary patient. I conclude he'll be difficult to intubate, but perhaps not all that difficult. I can try to get the tube in after he goes to sleep. Intubating someone with a difficult airway while they're still awake and breathing spontaneously is usually the safer course, but it's more stressful. I worry how much stress Charlie can take.

I sit down next to Charlie for a talk. I tell him what will happen, what his experience will be like from this moment forward. I describe the operating room and who will be in it, the monitors I'll be using, and what it will be like for him as he goes to sleep and wakes up.

I do this routinely with every patient, laying out options and recommendations, varying my description depending on circumstances. With Charlie, for example, I mention going to ICU afterward with a breathing tube in place. I also try a little humor on him, my attempt to dispel tension:

"We make the operating room look the way it does on TV. And everyone wears pajamas."

"Okay," he says, not smiling.

Some patients don't want to know anything (just put me out), and with those I keep it short. But I always end with the same words to everyone:

I'll never leave you while you're asleep. I'll be watching over you the whole time. But you won't have any sense of time passing. You won't believe when it's over. When you wake, you'll be asking when it's going to start.

Charlie doesn't ask about risks. By law I'm supposed to explain them, but this is tricky because no law is subtle enough to provide universal guidance. There are thousands of things we know of that can go wrong with an anesthetic and probably thousands more that nobody has dreamed of.

Anesthesia is a lot safer now than it was fifty years ago, and the chance of dying from an anesthetic is very small, perhaps one in 200,000. But statistics can prove most anything depending on how you manipulate them. What I really want to do is convey a sense of gravity and safety at the same time.

I often tell patients that lightning can always strike, but the most dangerous part of the day is driving to the hospital. This is sort of true, depending on what you mean by danger. I mention common side effects and complications, and then I ask, "Do you want me to explain specifically about all the risks?"

Almost invariably the answer is no.

With Charlie it's a little different. His anesthetic is going to be a lot more dangerous than a car ride and he needs to know it.

"I must tell you," I say to him, "that putting you to sleep carries a real risk to your life."

"I know," he says, looking straight into my eyes.

We leave it at that.

        🐾 🐾 🐾

It's 6:55 a.m. and the OR is humming as doctors, nurses, orderlies, technicians and other staff glide through the corridors in their freshly cleaned scrubs accomplishing the myriad tasks of preparation. Computers must be consulted, patients located and sent for, supplies ordered and counted, instruments picked and sterilized, and equipment assembled and checked. And forms, endless forms, paid homage.

I head for room four, my home for the day. I arrive before the nurses. The space is a study in white—smooth white walls and ceiling, white bulletin boards, white linoleum floor, white surgical lamps, white X-ray panels, and white built-in counter tops. Against that angelic background, the flat panel video screens suspended from above float darkly.

Two pieces of equipment particularly concern me: my cart and the anesthesia machine. The cart looks like a red mechanic's cart in an auto shop—a series of drawers topped by flat counter space—except it's clean and ocean blue. It travels with me wherever I'm assigned a case, and I've decorated it with a couple of pictures of my son.

The anesthesia machine lives in the room and, though on wheels, never moves much. It's designed to do one thing: deliver a mixture of oxygen and anesthetic gas. A metal/glass conglomeration of vaporizers, flow meters, ventilator, and hoses, it towers over the other equipment, an oddly-shaped spacecraft.

Together, cart and machine are my chief allies, my safety net, my refuge. I maneuver them to create an enclosed space for myself at the head of the operating table where I can view the procedure over the ether screen.

This is anesthesia territory, a closet-size bit of real estate over which I am sovereign, and here I'll spend most of my day. I won't spend much time observing surgery, however. The anesthesia machine has a metal shelving system on which sit an array of screens displaying patient data—respiration, oxygenation, EKG, blood pressure, and so forth, and it's these I'll be concerned with once the case gets going.

The cart contains drugs and equipment for the case. What you need for every contingency—every possible disaster that can strike—you want within easy reach on your cart. If a patient goes into a death spiral before your eyes you can't leave the room to hunt for something or be rummaging through drawers. It must be in a state of readiness, precisely where you left it, unmoved and untouched by other hands.

I check the machine to make sure it's functioning properly, and then set out on the cart what I'll need—all the tools my plan for Charlie requires. This takes some thought, and if I'm early, as I am today, I'll be alone in the room for a few minutes and can work without distraction.

At 7:15 a.m. the circulating nurse arrives with Charlie on a gurney. I look over my checklist to be sure I've left nothing out and we move him to the OR table. Most patients can shimmy over by themselves, but we need to use a slider to help Charlie.

"Did you get your shot?" I say to him.

I've prescribed morphine to relax Charlie and atropine to dry his mouth. His airway is worry enough without saliva getting in the way.

"Yeah. My mouth's pretty dry," he says between labored breaths. "Can I get a beer?"

I hand him a cup with a quarter ounce of water in it.

"Swish it around," I say. "That will be $10,000."

Charlie grins and downs it in one gulp.

Anesthesia requires an empty stomach, but a little water at the last minute isn't going to hurt.

I inspect Charlie's IV for kinks—it needs to run like a fire hose. I select a blood-pressure cuff that will fit Charlie's huge arm, then flip a switch to inflate it. I have a manual cuff on my cart if I need it, but I'm hoping the automated device will do the job—one less task to divert me during the case. The cuff works. I fit an oxygen mask over Charlie's face, making sure of the seal.

"You need to breathe pure oxygen for five to ten minutes before going to sleep," I say.

Anesthesia masks make some patients claustrophobic. They make me claustrophobic. In an uncomplicated case I can wait until the patient is asleep to apply the mask. But Charlie will have to suffer through it no matter what. I want every cell in his body saturated with 100 percent oxygen, which buys me precious time if his airway proves difficult. A person who has been breathing room air can hold his breath about a minute.

Someone who has been breathing pure oxygen for five minutes can go two or three times longer.

Fortunately Charlie is used to masks and accepts it without complaint.

"Time-out?" says the nurse.

Of all the regulations imposed on operating rooms, "time-outs" make the most sense. The time-out is a pre-flight check designed to make sure everyone is ready to proceed, and to prevent wrong limb surgery, wrong patient surgery, allergic reactions and other avoidable mistakes. When the time-out is called everything stops and a checklist is consulted. Everyone in the room must agree on the answers, including the patient, before the case can proceed.

There are actually two time-outs, one before anesthesia starts and one before the incision. Some OR staff grumble about overkill but someday I would like to thank personally the genius who insisted on a separate time-out for anesthesia.

It's not the enforced checklist that makes me grateful; I have my own checklist anyway. I love the pre-anesthesia time-out because it means no one can rush me into starting a case. If I say I'm not prepared for the time-out, the time-out waits.

"Time-out," I say.

☙ ☙ ☙

Readiness is all. It's zero hour for Charlie and me. I've

decided not to intubate him while he is awake—I fear the stress on him will be too great. One way or another I believe I can get a breathing tube into Charlie's trachea after he's asleep, and I have backup plans if this proves impossible.

Getting Charlie to sleep will require a big dose of induction agent. I plan to use both Pentothal and propofol on him, a lot of Pentothal and propofol.

"How are you going to poison him, Tiger?" one of my attending professors, a man almost as large as Charlie, used to ask me when we'd meet to discuss a case beforehand.

Poison indeed. When the induction agents hit Charlie's brain, the respiratory center will temporarily shut down and he'll stop breathing. Once again, I imagine myself and my patient in a small boat poised at the top of a waterfall, a long drop to the rocks below us.

"Should I count?" Charlie asks as I turn up the IV.

"If you like," I say, "But as long as you're awake, take nice even breaths."

Patients often feel they should count or count backwards, because they've seen it in movies. I suppose the purpose, apart from the drama, is to announce unconsciousness as the counting trails off. But a deep sigh, closing of the eyes, and loss of the blinking reflex does as well for me.

Charlie closes his eyes and takes one big breath, his last for the time being. The induction drugs have reached his respiratory center. I brush my finger against his eyelash; no blink. The pulse oximeter reads 100 percent saturation—he's been breathing pure oxygen for seven minutes.

I squirt ointment in his eyes and tape them closed, then slip a small plastic airway into his mouth to keep his tongue from falling back into his throat. I extend his neck and grip the mask hard in my left hand, hooking a finger behind his jawbone to push it forward. I find the anesthesia bag with my right hand, ready to squeeze. I say a prayer.

I've reached a fork in the road. If I can force air into Charlie's lungs at this point, that is, if I can ventilate him by mask, then I can proceed with the intubation attempt. But if I can't—if Charlie's chest doesn't rise and fall with each squeeze of the bag—it means that I'm probably pushing oxygen through the esophagus into his stomach where it does no good.

This was the point I got into trouble with Sam— proceeding with the intubation attempt when I couldn't ventilate by mask. It's not a mistake I ever intend to make again.

If I can't ventilate Charlie with the mask, I'll quickly put in a laryngeal mask airway. I have one ready on my cart. Charlie's tissue is now so saturated with oxygen that I should be able to accomplish this long before he starts turning blue. At least that's the theory.

If I can't ventilate Charlie with the LMA, I'll allow him

to wake up. Once he's breathing on his own again we can move on to a different plan, probably the awake intubation.

Assuming I can ventilate Charlie, I'll follow that by giving Anectine, the same muscle relaxant I used with Sam. The generic name for Anectine is succinylcholine ("sux" for short), and despite the trouble it gave me with Sam, I consider it one of the most useful drugs in my arsenal.

When I was a kid my favorite set of books was a science fiction series, *Tom Corbett, Space Cadet*, which unfolded 300 years from now. Tom's imagined future sported some impressive merchandise, chief among them his weapon, the *parlo ray*. If Tom hit you with a blast from his parlo ray your body would freeze; your muscles would stay frozen until a negative blast reversed the paralysis.

Sux does roughly the same thing, except that it knocks out the muscles of breathing in the bargain, which apparently a parlo ray did not. Sux is rapidly metabolized by an enzyme in the blood (another departure from the parlo ray) and wears off faster than any other muscle relaxant, which is why I like it. But the time it takes a body to recover from sux is still outside the four-minute window of safety.

How lovely it would be to have a drug that produced complete paralysis for only a minute or two. Alas, such an agent doesn't exist.

I set aside these thoughts for the moment, and let my hands do my thinking for me. Unconsciousness has softened the muscles around Charlie's neck and I can get a good feel for how difficult an airway he has. His skin is cold and slightly clammy. I press inward, testing the resiliency of the tissue. My hands confirm my earlier judgment: it won't be easy to get the tube through the vocal cords and into the trachea, but I should be able to do it.

I squeeze the bag. Charlie's chest rises—I can ventilate him.

Onward.

Charlie's surgery—a femoral artery repair—is not one that demands an endotracheal tube. But general anesthesia on its own will depress breathing, and Charlie is already close to respiratory failure. He needs to be mechanically ventilated during the case, for which a breathing tube is ideally suited.

Could the operation be done with a spinal anesthetic—keeping Charlie pain free, awake, and breathing on his own? I doubt it. He'll be lying flat for the procedure, and I think his breathing would get progressively worse during the case. I reckon that ultimately he would end up needing to be tubed anyway—and under urgent conditions. Better now, when I have leisure.

I give the Anectine.

The drug flows through the IV into the bloodstream, which distributes it quickly to muscle cells throughout Charlie's body. In response, his muscles begin to contract, which I can see as little twitches all over his frame. It's as if his muscles are taking one last bow before retiring from the stage. This effect of Anectine may give Charlie muscle cramps tomorrow, which he won't thank me for.

The twitching starts to subside. Until the Anectine wears off, Charlie's diaphragm can't contract again.

Even with relaxation it's hard squeezing the reservoir bag against Charlie's bulk. It's hard holding the anesthesia mask in position. It won't be long before the flexors in my forearm tire and start to cramp. They'll ache tomorrow along with Charlie's muscles.

But I'm relieved at this point. At least I can ventilate him. If I don't get the tube in I can always go back to masking him until the sux wears off—maybe ten minutes from now—and he can breathe for himself.

Charlie's body stills. I insert a standard laryngoscope into his mouth over his tongue until the epiglottis—the flap of tissue that covers the vocal cords when you swallow food—comes into view.

It's a long way down, and as I lift the epiglottis I can't quite see Charlie's vocal cords underneath it, where they should be. The right-angled path is too severe. This is disappointing, and it means that I have another decision to make.

I can shove the tube in blindly now and hope for the best. But the tube may enter the esophagus, which is just behind the trachea. While not a disaster unless it's unrecognized by the anesthetist, an esophageal intubation would be a setback. And Charlie is not a good candidate for setbacks. With Charlie, I've got to be certain.

On my cart is a device called the AirTraq. This is a fiberoptic laryngoscope designed to see around the curves of a difficult airway. I had taken the precaution of lubricating one and loading in an endotracheal tube so it's ready to go if I need it.

It's at this point I notice a dismaying change in the pulse oximeter's tone. It starts to fall. Another glitch.

"What's the saturation?" I ask the nurse—I don't want to look up from Charlie's mouth.

"Ninety-five," she says.

I'd thought there would be time before Charlie started needing more oxygen. He had seven full minutes breathing 100 percent, apparently not long enough for the cells of his body. What to do? Remove the laryngoscope and ventilate more with the mask? What if I can't reverse the falling oxygen saturation? Try an LMA?

I'm still pretty sure I can get the AirTraq in, but what if I can't? Get help? Perhaps I should have asked another anesthesiologist to stand by just in case—if I had, he'd be here now. The plan, which had been so clear in my mind a moment ago, is now fuzzier.

Whatever you do, I tell myself, *do it quick and do it now.*

I can feel my own heart beating faster as I decide to try

one other trick before moving on to fiberoptics. With my standard laryngoscope still in place, I ask the circulating nurse to push gently down on Charlie's neck. The pressure nudges the vocal cords in my direction, and I can just make out the cartilage that supports them from behind. This tells me exactly where the cords ought to be.

I grab a stylet I'd also set out in advance—a long, thin, solid tube made of flexible plastic—and advance it through Charlie's mouth in the direction of the unseen vocal cords. It's still possible that the stylet could make its way into the esophagus. But as it advances I can feel it brushing against the rings of the trachea like a stick being dragged along a picket fence. The vibration tells me the stylet is where I want it to be.

Now I can pass the endotracheal tube over the stylet and into the trachea. Home free—except the tube snags on the vocal cords and won't pass farther.

"Eighty-four percent," says the nurse. The oxygen tones continue to fall.

The tube is too large, I tell myself. *You've used too large a tube*.

It will take time to prepare another. How much time do I have?

Everything slows. The boat has carried Charlie and me well over the falls. An uncanny, weightless feeling comes over me as I contemplate the rocks below. Sam again? Fey?

I twist the endotracheal tube, pushing as I do. The edge

of the tube is beveled, and there should be a point when it disengages from the vocal cords. Suddenly it gives. The fit is tight, but it passes into the trachea.

"Eighty percent," says the nurse.

I pull out the stylet and connect the tube to my anesthesia circuit. Then I squeeze the bag. I squeeze and squeeze and squeeze. The oxygen saturation falls to 73, and then begins to rise.

From here on the sailing gets smoother.

"Oh, you're tubing him," says the surgeon, walking in. "You're going to pull it when we're done, right?"

"Not a chance," I say. "You probably noticed his respiratory failure."

"Whatever you say, doc."

By now I've attached Charlie to the ventilator, which will be breathing for him. I dial on a vaporizer, which adds anesthetic gas to the oxygen already in the circuit. I listen with a stethoscope for breath sounds—gas whooshing in and out of Charlie's lungs. There would be none if the tube was in Charlie's esophagus. But I can hear the sounds of ventilation faintly on both sides of Charlie's chest through layers of fat. His oxygen saturation is 85 percent and climbing.

One more test to be sure of the tube's position: I hook a capnograph into the breathing circuit to measure the concentration of carbon dioxide.

As a result of normal metabolic process the body

produces a small amount of carbon dioxide that is exhaled through the lungs with every breath. This continues even in an anesthetized body. A tube in the trachea will have carbon dioxide from the lungs in it, and a tube in the esophagus won't.

Charlie's capnograph tracing is normal, which means the breathing tube is positioned right on the money. The concentration of carbon dioxide also tells me how well Charlie is being ventilated. If the concentration is too high, it means the carbon dioxide in the lungs isn't being sufficiently cleared out. I increase the rate and volume of ventilation until I'm satisfied. The oxygen saturation hits 90, still climbing.

￼ ￼ ￼

The hardest part of my day is now over. I have three more assigned cases, but they loom as mere ponds next to Charlie's Sargasso Sea.

The technical difficulty of his intubation turned out to be only moderate. What made it nerve-racking were his weight and respiratory problems and the unexpectedly small size of his trachea. As far as I'm concerned the sight of his chest rising and falling is one of the marvels of nature.

Charlie's body surrenders easily, almost gratefully to mechanical ventilation. I'll leave the breathing tube in after the case, as I planned. When Charlie is fully awake and all his other post-operative problems are under control, perhaps later today, perhaps tomorrow morning, the lung specialist can remove the tube (extubate) with Charlie's feedback and cooperation.

The nurses can prep and drape now and the surgeon proceed with his business. On my side of the drapes I arrange things to suit myself. It's a habit of mine to keep a part of the body in my field of view at all times—in this instance Charlie's head—as a reality check on what my instruments are telling me. A throwback, I suppose, to W. T. G. Morton and the early days when there were no anesthesia instruments, not even a blood pressure cuff, just the anesthetist's hand on the pulse.

I wouldn't want to have given anesthesia in Morton's day. Since his time, the rates of complication and death from anesthesia have steadily lowered. That makes me grateful for my modern anesthesia pharmacy, for all my electronic monitoring, my fiberoptic and other clever airway devices, my sophisticated anesthesia machine.

I'm also thankful for Otto, Rose, Sam, and thousands of others for what they've taught me. I'm even more thankful they're still alive.

There will be other problems to solve as Charlie's surgery progresses, other clinical decisions to make, but nothing as fraught as what Charlie and I have just passed through. There are even some respiratory tests I learned as a resident that I could perform at the end of the procedure. The results might indicate whether it would be safe to pull the tube out early.

I could push our luck and maybe get away with it—something I might have tried at the outset of my career.

But I'm not the person I was then.

ACKNOWLEDGMENTS

Cover art: Lorraine Bubar

Cover design: Jeff Smith

Title page illustration—Earnest Board, *The dentist William TG Morton*

Thanks to the following for reading and commenting on drafts of this book: Robert Massing, Steve Totland, Rena Copperman, John Sylvain, Graham Liebman, Larry Lang, and Carrie Cantor.

I am grateful to Dr. Michelle Au for her description of anesthesiologists as the last clinical generalists, which idea I incorporated into the prologue.

AFTERWARD

Thank you for purchasing this book. Word of mouth from reader to reader is critical to an author's success. If you enjoyed these pages, please consider leaving a review at the Amazon store.

To learn more about me or my writing, find me online at wolfpascoe.com, for the latest news or to contact me.

Wolf Pascoe

Made in the USA
Lexington, KY
14 June 2013